RECIPROCATED LOVE:

THE HEART of a CAREGIVER

by Camille (Cam) Carter

Copyright © 2023

All rights reserved.

No part of this book may be reproduced in any form for any reason without expressed written permission from author.

ACKNOWLEDGEMENTS

My Sons (J & Q): As humans, we each reach our Life's purpose at varying intervals, various time-frames, and whenever that "appointed" time is, for each of us. As parents, this realization makes it so, that you are constantly growing; learning; improving; and Ultimately, becoming the Best versions of 'Yourselves'. Now, young Men, Your responsibility is to apply the Humility; Morals; Qualities; and Values into your own lives, that your Father and I instilled into Both of you. As self-development guru, Dean Graziosi says, "Life is about KAIZON...**Progress**, NOT perfection." And as Your mama, I Thank God for choosing Me to Mother You and I Love You Both, endlessly.

My Grandchildren (A & Q): It's an Honor, to have been there for both of your births and to watch you Both grow up and thrive. I feel Tremendously BLESSED, that I was hand-picked by God, to be a Grandma to the two (2) of You. I feel Great JOY and Immense Pleasure, knowing that You two (2) are a part of My lineage and legacy. Grandma Loves You very much!

Mother of My Grandchildren (M.T.): Shout-out for being an Awesome mother to my Grandbabies. Thank YOU!

The first (1st) of many More books, projects, etc. to come and God-willing, You're there like you've remained, right by My side. ALWAYS Encouraging; Supportive; Positively optimistic; and reminding Me, that I can do Anything with God's help. So Yes, may the 'REAL Joe' stand up, please? To You, J: My Soulmate; the Best Friend a girl could EVER have; My Prayer Warrior King; My 'Better' Half; My Man- the ONLY Man I want to do this thing called life (with); My Ying (to My Yang); and ALLLLL the 'Good' stuff in-between....*My Husband.* Thank You for being YOU and who God made you to be, for ME. I am so absolutely Appreciative and Grateful for Our Union; Our Bond; Our Friendship; Our Relationship; Our Marriage; Our Commitment; Our Laughter....US! Hats off, I Salute You. I Love You.

And last, but NOT least, to the *Ones* who prayed; uplifted; encouraged; helped (in any way); etc. during My Caregiving journey-'Thank You' from the bottom of My heart: *My Mama, J.H.; My Aunt, L.J.; former Step-dad, W.H.; former Church-Family @ G.A. in Tulsa, OK (especially Pastors S.B. & Sister D.B. (RIP); Mrs. T.M.; Ms. Ber and Many others but too many to name); Family-Friends P.M. (RIP) & T.M.; G.H. & R.H.; C.M.; K.B.; and Soul-Sister, T.M.* xoxo

DEDICATION

This book is Dedicated to the '**Real**' Angels-'2 of the 3', who made an indomitable impact in My life, as they did with countless others. May you BOTH Rest in HARMONIOUS Peace, for Infiniti....*My Grandma, Ms. B.F.L. and My Mother-in-Law, Ms. JoE.C.*

TABLE OF CONTENTS

INTRODUCTION 8

ACT 1: My Grandma's Story 10
   CHAPTER 1: Yep, That's Her! My Grandma,
   Ms. Bertie Lewell 12
   CHAPTER 2: A Ray of Sunshine 15
   CHAPTER 3: I'd Rather Be a Good Person 17
   CHAPTER 4: Party of Five (5) 19
   CHAPTER 5: Healthy Lifestyle 22
   CHAPTER 6: More than Physical Needs 25
   CHAPTER 7: Unequivocally and Unconditionally 27
   CHAPTER 8: God Doesn't Make (Any) Mistakes ... 30
   When Caring for a Chronically Ill Loved One: 32
   Healthcare Professionals for Caregivers: 34

ACT 2: Joe's Story 36
   CHAPTER 1: The Beginning, Joe Carver Sr. 38
   CHAPTER 2: Life Goes On and On & On and On 41
   CHAPTER 3: It Is, What It Is 44
   CHAPTER 4: But God 46
   CHAPTER 5: About that Life 51

ACT 3: Ms. Carver's Story **54**
   CHAPTER 1: No News Is Good News 56
   CHAPTER 2: The Fragile State of Life............................58
   CHAPTER 3: At the End of the Day................................61
   CHAPTER 4: The Matriarch..65
   CHAPTER 5: Dignity, Love, and Respect:
   FULL STOP..67
   CHAPTER 6: Never…Ever..69
   CHAPTER 7: Remembered, Always...................................71
   Caring for a Hospice Care Patient or
   Incapacitated Loved One: 73

INTRODUCTION

The stories that I've shared, that are Dear to my heart and what you'll be reading, partaking in something that I'm truly Passionate about-it means a lot to me. I've known for a while that I wanted, but most importantly needed, to share my experiences (ALL of them) about caregiving. More directly, 'My Tribe'-the people who this will resonate with the most. Whether you are currently a Caregiver or are on the cusp of becoming one, I graciously understand your plight. It is something that is not always understood or often an endeavor that is overlooked, but rewarding, nevertheless. Above all, I would change nothing, regarding the lives I've given my care and unwavering love to…absolutely NOTHING. They have each affected and enriched my life in so many different and various ways, that I'm Grateful for our many interactions. I'm teary-eyed, as I write and remember, 'The Three'. 'The Three' of a few, whom I will Forever love, cherish, and respect-that entrusted Me with their Care, their lives. And I did so with great Pride and Honor. In essence, that is what is at the core of "giving care" in caregiving. Someone believing in another, to help them navigate their wellness; healthcare; well-being; etc. Being proactive on their health journey, as well as, their advocate. During each experience, I learned a multitude of things like Dos and Don'ts, while being a Caregiver and I'd like to share them with You. I'm aware while taking care of someone-it's not like you're given a map, a guide, or even a manual. Therefore, at times, you're learning and "doing" by trial and error. In my case, I have a background in Medical front office procedures. I was in the field for many years involving Patient Accounts Specialist; Medical billing; Insurance verifications; Pre-invoice verifications; and Physician's & Hospital billing practices. Because I'd been around doctors; nurses; medical assistants; et cetera.-I'd picked up a lot of Intel, which would later become beneficial. It's like that saying, "Chew up what you can use and spit out the rest, that doesn't apply." (DISCLAIMER: I am NOT medically certified and/or trained to treat, diagnose, et-cetera Anyone, then or now). So thankfully, when it became necessary for me to be a Caregiver for my Grandma, my Husband, and my Mother-in-law ('The Three', in the order in which I cared for them), I had some knowledge, of what to do, and where to start. However, if you're new to caregiving, please do NOT be discouraged, because you have the Main pre-requisite as a Caregiver: Love AND Compassion. Further, NO amount of schooling or formal training can teach you, what is in your Soul. So having the Heart & Empathy, to 'Step-In and Step-Up' for Someone in your life...Yes, YOU are Enough. Yes, YOU can do this too (virtual hug)! And I hope that My story offers Help to you in the care of your loved one(s). More than anything, ALWAYS lead with your Heart as I did.

***DISCLAIMER**: Although this book, along with these stories are based on **True accounts** & **Real individuals** (Dead and Alive), they are from My own POV (Point of View) and Personal experiences. Further, out of *Respect and Privacy* for my Family, ALL names have been changed. *

ACT 1

My Grandma's Story

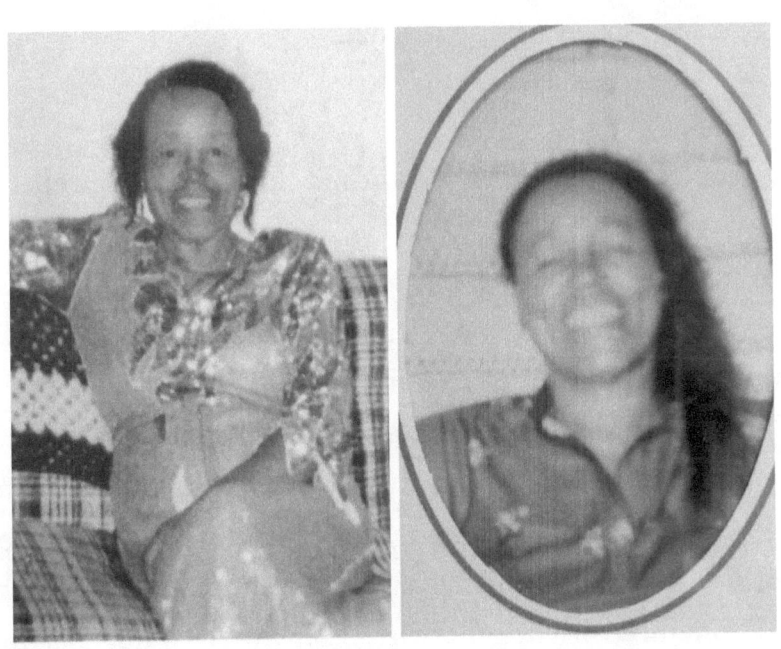

My Beautiful Grandma, Ms. B.F.L.

CHAPTER 1:

Yep, That's Her! My Grandma, Ms. Bertie Lewell

Ms. Bertie Lewell, the first (1st) of 'The Three' (3) was Honorable; Trustworthy; Dependable; Sincere; Upright…I could go on and on to describe my Grandma. During my adolescence, I looked at and up to her, as the 'Blueprint' of life. I mean sure, I knew she was only Human. Just a woman, who consisted of blood; bones; flesh, and skin-just like you and me. As a child, my naiveté wasn't such, that my psyche had convinced itself, otherwise. I was well aware, that this Wonderful Human being was simply a mere mortal and her life had an expiration date, like everyone else's. However, I had <u>ALWAYS</u> viewed 'Madear and Mama' (what her children still call her)-my Grandma, as the 'Epitome' of who a Christian was and should be. Whether male or female. Fondly called 'Sis Lewell', by those who knew and admired her. And as Pretty; as Captivating; as Gorgeous; as Angelic and as Strikingly-beautiful as I recognized my Grandma to be on the exterior-

her Kindness; Ardor; Heart; Character; Spirit and Aura, matched the interior. She embodied Godly and intangible traits, that could NEVER be procured or acquired. What she possessed internally, well they were absolutely Priceless and God-given. In my eyes, this is 'Who' my Grandma was and what she meant to Me. I Loved <u>EVERYTHING</u> about this enchanting beauty-God's extraordinary creation. Ms. Bertie or 'Sis Lewell', was the type of individual, that if you wronged her, she'd "turn the other cheek" and then pray for you. Without any malice or ill-intentions, my Grandma would Genuinely pray for your forgiveness AND your salvation. I've witnessed this very thing, while growing up under my Grandma's care. I can recall an incident, as a young kid. I may have been either five (5) or six (6) years of age and we had recently moved into a city housing development, back in the early 80's. Apparently, when my Mama, June and her siblings had dropped off a load of household items at our "new" residence, someone forgot to lock the backdoor at the apartment. So when they came back to drop off an additional load, they noticed that the backdoor was left wide open and unattended! Many of my Grandma's personal belongings were missing and some, irreplaceable. One of the aforementioned, was my Grandfather Jamie's Military flag that my Grandma received as his widow, after his death. There were quite a few items that had been burglarized. I just remember my Mama, June; my Aunt Liz; and my Uncle Dalen being really Angry and Upset. My mama was HOT, absolutely Furious! Then somehow, they found this woman, who had some of my Grandma's personal property inside of her car trunk. The stolen goods DEFINITELY belonged to her, because on the back of each item were my Grandma's initials and in HER Own handwriting! Eventually, the woman pointed my Mama and her siblings, to the Actual culprits of the robbery and where she'd paid for the "hot" (stolen) merchandise. However, before anyone could react or retaliate, my Grandma stepped-in and intervened. I don't recall the exact conversation or precisely what was said, but I do remember her praying about the situation. On her knees later that night, my Grandma asked God to forgive them and prayed that they'd "come to know Him." YEP, that was My Grandma alright, Sister Lewell! Now do you see why I adored her, so much? She was like a Real-life, living and breathing Angel, here on Earth.

CHAPTER 2:

A Ray of Sunshine

My Grandma and I were fifty (50) years apart, in age. By the time that I was born, she'd been alive for half (1/2) a century. In all of those years, surely Grandma had experienced many facets of life-the good and the not-so, but she'd always remained humbled and an optimist. I'd never heard her complain or get down on herself, even if life was indeed, "kicking her butt". She always had a sunny disposition and a friendly demeanor. Often, Grandma would portray a broad smile, exposing her dimpled cheeks. 'Sis Lewell' was just a cheerful person, who had an amazingly gleeful personality and attitude, very hospitable. She even loved sports like baseball and football, especially the Atlanta Braves. She understood the "ins and outs" of both sports, too. I'm sure some of her knowledge came from when her son, my Uncle Dalen played each sport. Grandma once shared with me, that she liked Hall of Famer, Mr. Emmett Smith because, "he did A Lot for his hometown of Pensacola, Florida", when he was a Dallas Cowboy. She'd moved there years earlier with my Aunt Shannon, when I was still in elementary school.

Pensacola became her home for many years, until years later when she moved back to her hometown in Oklahoma. She liked that about Mr. Smith. I can't say if she was a "Dallas Cowboy" fan or not, but Grandma admired the philanthropy work, that he did within his community. So, I guess that saying is true, "It takes one, to know one" and it applied to her. Because when I was growing up, she would frequently and freely give of herself, by giving back. Ofttimes, Grandma would do so in multiple and various ways. 'Sis Lewell' was a DEFINITE Class act, a real Lady. And she Always put people First (1), regardless of the situation. Those early lessons taught me a lot in life. It allowed me, to consciously apply them in my own adulthood, as a married woman with children.

CHAPTER 3:

I'd Rather Be a Good Person

Throughout my Grandma's life, she'd been heavily active and fully involved in church (choir; mission; usher staff; Leader/President on various boards, and traveling to hundreds of conventions). She attended and completed courses at a Bible Institution, graduating with an emphasis in Theology and Biblical studies. She also mentored both children and young adults. My Grandma was a well-rounded individual, who could get along with Anyone. Obviously attractive and very pretty, she **NEVER** obsessed over her outer beauty or looks. Although Ms. Bertie was Definitely "a looker", it didn't phase her and she concentrated on being a 'Good' person, instead. She cared about Humanity and the Goodwill of others. Though not vain in the least, she took care of herself with what she consumed. Grandma lived the motto, "The body is a temple and should not be defiled", Biblical law (paraphrase). She loved to walk, as a form of low-intensity exercise. While talking to her on the phone when she resided in Florida, she'd share her weekly fitness schedule with me. Grandma would walk around the mall in 2-3 intervals, several times per week. In her 70s at the time, it always amazed me how active she still was. Overall, Sis Bertie was a Genuinely jovial woman. As the current saying goes, "If treat your neighbor (Kindly), as yourself were a person"-it would have DEFINITELY been My Grandma, 'Sister Bertie Lewell'! *smile* The outer meant absolutely nothing to her because she purposefully concentrated on the Person. Her concern was about the soul and the Human spirit, itself.

CHAPTER 4:

Party of Five (5)

Ms. Bertie Lewell was the Mother of nine (9) children and interestingly enough, she was the baby girl/daughter out of nine (9) children. By the time I came into the world, my Grandma had five (5) living children, one of which included my mama. And as a young woman, 'Sis Bertie' became the Caretaker to her Mother, Mama Heinz. She was also a Grandmother, who made unselfish sacrifices and raised me. In essence, my Grandma was my 'Caregiver' as a child and she loved me, Unconditionally. The lineage of a Faithful, unwavering Prayer Warrior, who was truly a Devoted, Devout, and Honest woman of God. So when my Grandma's health began failing, I wanted to be able to repay her, for a lifetime of 'Her' generosity. One who poured into my life, consistently. I wanted to Honor her and for me, it was just that. A true Honor. It was a privilege and one that I definitely did NOT take lightly. So, first things first, after praying about the situation-I needed to have a conversation with my Husband, Joe. Over the years, we had developed a systems of sorts. We would discuss whatever was on the "agenda" then make an informed and sensible decision, together. Before I could state everything in its entirety or make any specific plans, Joe informed me that we were on the same page. In regards to my Grandma's health and being responsible for her care full-time, my Husband shared that our sentiments were in sync. He knew the depths of my love for my Grandma and Joe loved her, just as much. So, arrangements were made and we became Grandma's Primary Caregivers. I had just turned twenty-nine (29) years old, a few months prior. I worked a full-time job that I enjoyed, as well as Joe. He and I had two (2) children, Quavi and Justin, who were in elementary and middle school. They both had packed schedules, that included multiple sports apiece (baseball; basketball; football; and soccer), volunteer obligations, and extra-curricular/after-school activities. Justin was in Red Cross; Student Council; Junior Achievements and an Arts program, while Quavi played saxophone in band and was in Boys Scouts. Further, Joe and I had an active married life. Consequently, concessions and compromises had to be made. We sat our two (2) sons down and explained to them both, that their 'Aunt Granny' (the name Grandma's younger grand's, great-grand's, and great-great-grand's called her) would be moving in with us Full-time. They were both ecstatic, especially our youngest son, Justin. So shortly after our 'Family Meeting', Grandma came to live with my family and I. I had quit my job prior to her coming home, so the transition was a smooth and seamless one. And though slightly nervous, we couldn't have been more Excited. It was official, we were now a 'Party of Five' (5)!

CHAPTER 5:

Healthy Lifestyle

Remember living with Grandma during my childhood, I wanted her to feel comfortable and embrace all the love we could provide. As a result, it would require the entire household to be "all hands on deck". Therefore, in everything that we did, Grandma was always included. It was special, and a remarkable time for us. We cherished those moments, being able to bond with Grandma and the kids, their 'Aunt Granny'. At that junction, she was almost eighty (80) years old, so each shared occasion meant something...they were sacred. And though she'd been using a wheelchair for assistance and was nearly bedridden, it was of high importance to us, that Grandma had some semblance of her former self (before becoming ill). So, at the forefront of any business, was to safely decrease the number of medicines she'd been prescribed. Because it could be catastrophic, to immediately stop taking certain medications (especially for a Senior citizen), I knew this process would have to be Physician-led. Ultimately, I wanted her to be completely taken off <u>All</u> of her prescriptions, if possible. Since the '80s, my Grandma took a 'Naturally Organic' approach to her health and wellness. She ate a mainly plant-based diet with the occasional ground turkey, along with consuming ONLY supplements, vitamins, and/or minerals. As a matter of fact, she introduced me to vitamins and Omega-3's as a kid and I very rarely got sick. Moreover, Grandma drank ONLY purified water that had been previously boiled and then cooled, and on rare occasions, Crystal Light. This was years, long before bottled water had become as popular, as it is today. She'd been on this regime for quite some time and well into her early to mid-70s. Because I also recalled, experienced, and knew who she'd been during My lifetime-I wanted to gradually incorporate a 'Holistic' (healing) diet, back into her daily life. A lifestyle for optimal health, to revive and rejuvenate her on this wellness journey. Since I wasn't a doctor (then or now) nor certified to medically treat anyone, it was imperative to research professionals. We needed those, that could assist us in the course of maintaining my Grandma's healthcare. As I mentioned earlier, in the intro, I have a background in Medical billing and insurance, so that knowledge was valuable in finding the appropriate specialists and Medical personnel. I did my due diligence, to gather a 'Team' around her care. Since she was over the age of sixty-five (65), I knew it was paramount to choose a **good** 'Geriatric Primary Care Provider/Physician' (specializes in elderly patients, 65+), in her overall healthcare plan. Further, it had been a while at that point, since Grandma had been on a plant-based diet and she now had dietary restrictions. Therefore, a 'Registered Dietician' was necessary, because they're trained in food and nutrition. My Grandma was always a very active and vibrant woman who had an engaging and magnetic personality. Her presence was warm, dynamic, and inviting. So, a 'Physical Therapist' was a *MUST*, to assist in her mobility, and slowly get her active, again, at her own pace. Lastly, I needed a 'Certified Nursing Assistant' (CNA), to help me during the day, until my Husband came home after work. I didn't want to have to depend on anyone with these day-to-day tasks. I took my role seriously, as well as full responsibility for being Grandma's Primary Caregiver. I knew I could call on my Mama, but she'd had back surgery the previous year and was still in recovery. Furthermore, if need be, I could also contact my Uncle Dalen and his wife, Aunt Reba, as well as my Aunts Glory-Jan and Aunt Liz. My Aunt Shannon had planned to move Grandma back to Florida with her, once she completed college and moved back into a house. But I decided early on, to only contact my Aunts and/or Uncle due to an EMERGENCY or if my Husband and I absolutely could not do something. So Joe and I worked together, to incorporate a schedule that was feasible for our entire household. We had a plan in place, for the improvement of my Grandma's health. Shortly thereafter, Joe and I began our caregiving journey. We were then on our way!

CHAPTER 6:

More than Physical Needs

I knew this would be a long and tedious process-one that required patience, diligence, and fortitude. It was okay because I was completely dedicated and committed, to do whatever was necessary, according to my Grandma's health and medical capabilities. Above all, as long as SHE was comfortable, knew she was loved, and felt cared for, that was the Main priority. Since I no longer worked outside of the home, I'd care for Grandma while Joe went to work and our children were in school. Joe would get up earlier in the mornings and get everyone situated. He'd feed Grandma and our boys, while I took that time to get some extra rest. On some mornings, I'd hear Joe say, "Good Morning pretty Lady, how're You?" I'd giggle when Grandma would return with, "Good morning, pretty Lady" back to him. During this timeframe, it gave me an opportunity to relax, until it was time to care for my Grandma. Because I'd recalled how

'Intentional' she was about her daily activities, I introduced a regimen during our days together. For starters, she was avid in her Biblical reading and studying. Since a little girl, I have very fond and vivid memories of this. She'd start each and every morning in prayer; read her Bible; meditate on the 'Word' (the Holy Bible); and have quiet worship, while singing or humming a Hymnal to herself, BEFORE doing anything else. Then prior to retiring for the evening, I would join her for our nightly routine. We would get on our knees and pray, without fail. We would begin with the Lord's Prayer then Grandma would finish up by praying for Everyone ("the sick and shut-in"; our nation; our family; etc.). She was very specific in her prayers, including one for each of her five (5) living children. Those prayers were very Powerful and Heartfelt, forever cemented in my heart. As my Grandma's Caregiver, I would read the Bible to her. And she loved Gospel music! So oftentimes, I would play some in the background, while I prayed for and to her. These gestures were always apart of her day-to-day, so I wanted them to remain in her daily life. As an active Christian, Grandma's faith had always been a top priority. Therefore, along with making sure all of her physical necessities were met, it was **imperative** that Grandma's Spiritual and Soul needs were (met) too...

CHAPTER 7:

Unequivocally and Unconditionally...

Because my Grandma, 'Sister Lewell' was not actively using her legs without assistance at that time, the Certified Nursing Assistant (CNA) would help me during the daytime. It's been many years (early 2000's), so I don't remember the CNA's name, but she was very nice and a great asset. She would come 2-3 times per week, then assist me with basic and essential care needs for Grandma like baths; getting her up and dressed; taking vitals (temperature, blood pressure, pulse ox); etc. I never wanted my Grandma to feel burdensome and always attempted to make sure her Dignity remained intact. Because I never confused my role-my Grandma was STILL the adult and I would Forever treat her with the utmost care and respect. That was a NON-NEGOTIABLE factor. Before the CNA would leave for that day, she'd help me get Grandma in her wheelchair, then she and I would venture around our neighborhood. When the boys would come home from school, they'd do their homework, while Grandma napped and I would prepare dinner. Once Joe made it home from work, he'd take the boys to their sports practices if they had it. If not, we would spend Family time, after eating dinner then catch up on the day with everyone. Sometimes we would play a board game or watch T.V. together. Justin, our youngest son always wanted to be up under Grandma, kinda like me as a kid. Both of our boys would sit on either side of their 'Aunt Granny', while we watched television or played Monopoly, something of the sort. We developed a rhythm, our 'Family of Five' (5). And Grandma was in the mix of it all, soaking up all of our love and attention. Just thinking of her, recalling everything during that time, then writing this, I Miss My Grandma. But I'm comforted too because I have so many Wonderful memories with her and of her. When she lived in Florida, we always kept in touch. I still have letters, that she wrote to me with specific Bible scriptures for a multitude of things. We shared a lifetime of memorable moments, those that are filled with loads of laughter, tons of wisdom, and lots of savvy advice. All of which, that ONLY a Grandma could provide and offer. Truly Priceless! I'm reminiscent of when my Mama and I lived in South Carolina, with my Aunt Shannon and we'd drive to Florida to pick up Grandma. Since it was either Summertime or during the holidays, we would bring her back home with us to S.C. She would stay there for a few weeks before we'd take her back to Florida. While Aunt Shannon and Mama were at work during the daytime, Grandma and I would go to the mall, window-shopping. She and I would walk hand in hand, all around Northwoods Mall. At times, we'd run into classmates from my school and they would think that my nearly sixty (60) year old Grandma was my Mama! She did look as if she could have had a pre-teen because Grandma looked to be in her early 40s. It was funny, because "No" I'd say, "Actually, she's my Grandma" and she would just smile. I've been Blessed immensely because my Grandma is eternally in my heart. But more than anything, I'm Grateful that she knew that she was loved, Unequivocally and Unconditionally...

CHAPTER 8:

God Doesn't Make (Any) Mistakes

For the many years that my Grandma poured positively into my life and loved me, it was only fitting that she was credited with the same Honor. Always a giver, relentlessly kind-hearted, and forever thoughtful was Who she was. So she warranted our devotion and dedication. Unfortunately, we lost her right after her seventy-ninth (79) birthday, on March 08, 2003. Before things could be completely implemented to enrich her standard of life and prior to the fruition of my Grandma experiencing a "rebirth" of sorts, regarding her health, she expired. Died. That one (1) word was Hard to fathom, difficult to emotionally grasp. I'd <u>NEVER</u> thought of a time that my Grandma would not be here, on this earth, No matter her age or the situation. It has been nearly twenty (20) years, since her death and that pain has yet to dissipate, entirely. However, I hold onto the belief, that "God Doesn't make any mistakes", as she'd tell me. My Grandma lived her life and in her words, "to one day be with the Lord." Though not physically here any longer, I know she is in a "Better place, with her Lord and Savior, Jesus Christ", per My Grandma. So, I keep this one (1) sentiment close to My heart, that Grandma lived her life, as an Upright Christian and servant of Christ. She hadn't any qualms or fears about death, because her life had been in preparation for that very moment. My Grandma knew where her 'Forever Home' was, where she would reside for eternity, and with Whom. Therefore, it made the heartbreak of losing her just a little less hurtful. Just a smidgen; just a tiny bit; just an iota-less painful. But, not quite...

When Caring for a *Chronically Ill Loved One:*

(1) Asses your loved one's health condition(s)
A. Research the appropriate Professionals, regarding their 'Overall' health.
B. After doing your due diligence, interview and employ them, accordingly.
C. Assemble a 'Medical Team' (PCP, Specialist(s); Nutritionist; etc.) around their healthcare goals and/or needs.
D. Implement a 'Medical Plan', according to your loved one's health, along with their Physician(s).

(2) Be easy and Don't rush your loved one's process
A. Remember, do things according to 'Their' threshold and Medical Capabilities.
B. Take into account where your loved one is physically; mentally; emotionally; etc.
C. Be PATIENT, the course may be a slow & steady one.
D. Regardless where your loved one is on their Wellness journey, ALWAYS offer Encouragement.

(3) Always Remember-it is ALWAYS about them, your loved one-the *Recipient of Care*
A. Take your ego and emotions completely Out of the equation.
B. Decisions have to be made by You (the Caregiver), so your 'Heart♥Posture' needs to be pure.
C. It is NEVER about you, but the Betterment of your loved one and their Well-being & Health.

(4) Take time AWAY, If the situation is too difficult
A. Because your loved one may be Chronically-ill or be in crisis, Do NOT allow them to see you flustered or "feeling sorry for them or yourself".
B. NEVER make your loved one feel 'burdensome' or helpless.
C. 'Woo-saw' Breaks are okay (in intervals). Remember, YOUR actions, emotions, and reactions set the stage for the caregiving journey. Be Mindful of this…
D. The agenda should be to 'Improve' their Well-being and make them as Comfortable as possible, NOT 'regress' it. *I state this with the utmost, Sincerity*

Healthcare Professionals for Caregivers:

Listed below, are Medical professionals that were briefly mentioned during Ms. Bertie Lewell's story (My Grandma). They are each listed by title, along with a Detailed description of each profession.

<u>Geriatric Primary Care Provider/Physician</u> -Handles Non-emergency health issues and are the Main provider, for patients who are 65 years old or older.

<u>Registered Dietician</u>-Trained to counsel patients about food and nutrition. They have been 'Professionally' trained, to help with managing chronic illnesses.

<u>Nutritionist</u>-Teaches about food and nutrition. They help with meal plans, but are Not always registered (like a 'Registered Dietician').

<u>Physical Therapist</u>-Diagnoses the movements of patients and puts together a treatment plan.

<u>Certified Nursing Assistant (CNA)</u>-Does NOT have the official training of a Nurse, but are an integral part of a Medical team. They help with patients grooming; bathing; eating; mobility and work with patients who are bedridden (according to their own level of movement and dysfunction).

Source: **Google.com** *(I paraphrased each job profession, without changing the meaning and description of each one).*

ACT 2

Joe's Story

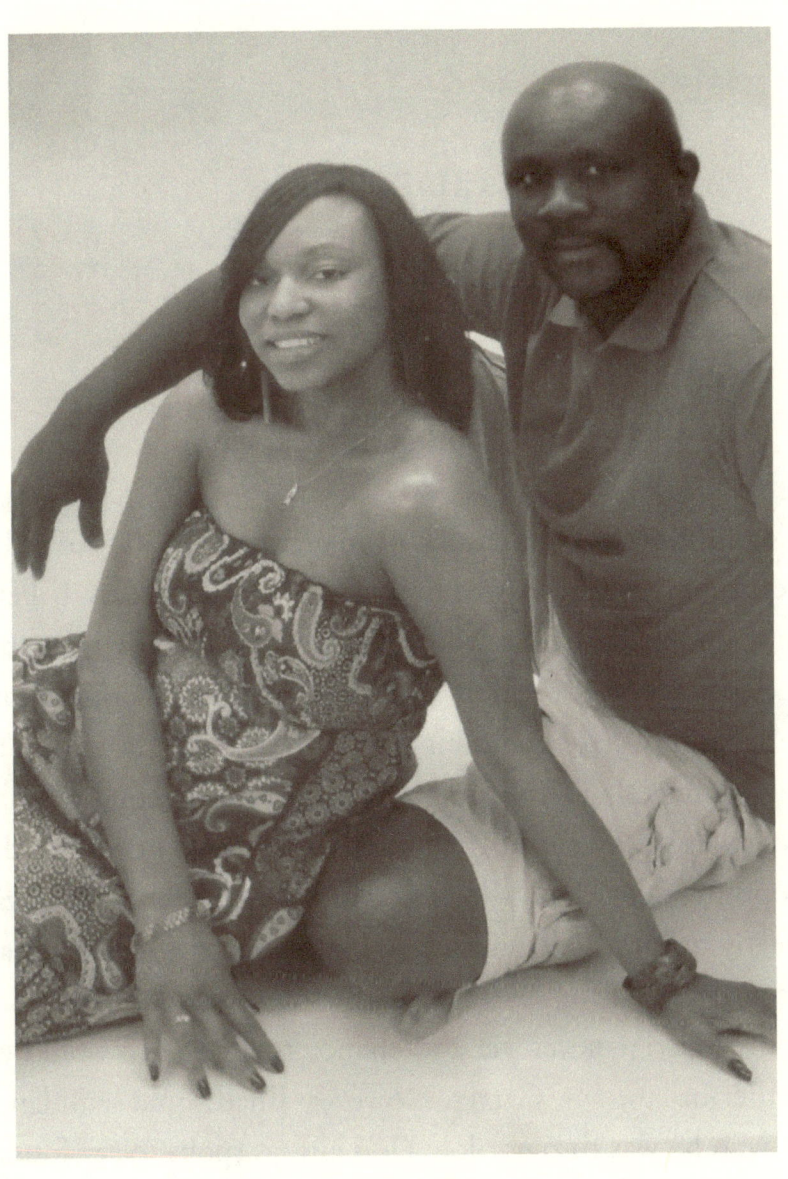

Me with My Hubby, J. Sr.

CHAPTER 1:

The Beginning, Joe Carver Sr.

No one is perfect, rather that be man or woman, boy or girl... perfection doesn't exist. However, I wholeheartedly believe that God made Joe for Me and I, for him. He is 'Perfect' for me, whatever 'Perfection' is. When we met, I noticed the relationship that he and his mother had. I paid attention to their interaction. It was definitely <u>not</u> in a creepy, "Mama's boy with an overbearing mother" kinda way, but quite the opposite. They had a loving 'Mother-Son' bond, that was clearly reciprocated, endearing. Unfortunately, Joe's dad had been deceased for several years, before he and I began our courtship. I'd never get the chance to meet my would-be Father-in-law, Mr. Carver. However, I had some semblance of who he was through Joe. He'd always spoken very fondly of Both of his parents-as individuals, as well as together, as a married couple. Listening to various stories from Joe and his Mom, Ms. Carver throughout the years, I was enthralled by their vivid and loving recollections. I enjoyed hearing them and other family members talk about the past and the "good ol days". But more than anything, I loved to witness the dynamic between Mother and son, even more. Their interaction was Always so easygoing, so laid back. The mutual respect and affection shared amongst the two (2) was truly heartwarming. I never felt "out of place", but rather embraced within the confines of their 'Mother-Son' relationship. It was just as easy, to fall in love with my now husband, Joe. Besides being extremely handsome and as they say "A tall glass of water", he had remarkable traits, as a man. It was obvious he loved his Mama, but he also had a quiet confidence; was real mellow with a 'chill' personality; he was thoughtful and kind. Further, Joe was smart (BOTH of our sons have Excellent mathematical skills and neither received them from Me, LOL!); witty; and Extremely Patient. The Lord knew Joe would need the patience of Job, being married to me, HA! *smile* Overall, he was just a very Caring guy. Within a month of dating, we BOTH just 'knew'. I'd told my best friend at the time that, "Joe is going to be my husband, one day". In that same time frame, he had sat his Mother and I down then proceeded to say, "Millie is going to be my wife and I'm going to marry her, Mama". Ms. Carver calmly responded, "Okay, if this is your decision, then I Support you both".

True to his word, Joe proposed to me on Christmas Eve 1993 and we married the following year, in October. Marrying young, I had a lot to learn. Well actually, we Both did. But no matter what, we decided early on, that we were in it for the long-haul, with the good AND the bad. Unbeknownst to us, we would need that same love, confidence, and assurance years down the line, when Joe was injured then became ill. Because, the '**Real**' work would begun and 'In sickness and In health'...would become a reality. FORREAL!

CHAPTER 2:

Life Goes On and On & On and On...

You know that phrase, "You never know what you would do when the going gets tough."? Better yet, (maybe) those were 'My' sentiments at the time. At that junction, Joe and I had been married for eleven (11) years and had experienced the normal 'ebbs & flow' of marriage, along with some tremendously devastating heartaches. We'd lost many loved ones, some who were very dear to us. Just two (2) years before Joe had fallen ill, we had become Primary Caregivers to my Maternal Grandma, who we lost a short time later. Filled with overwhelming grief and complete devastation, my Husband and I attempted to go on, with this journey called 'life'. Actually, there were no other alternatives.....life happens and the trek continues-one day at a time, step by step. So that's what we continued to do, 'Live Life', while parenting our two (2) school-aged children. Our sons were thirteen (13) and nine (9) years old, respectively. Joe and I worked full-time outside of the home and we each had busy, active lives. Joe played in a Men's Basketball league at his job. He was also our children's Basketball Coach and sometimes, he assisted on their football and baseball teams. I would tease him, that he went to the games as a "spectator" and would Always wind up as a Coach! LOL! It NEVER failed, but Joe would just laugh. It was fine with him, because he got the chance to spend more time with our boys plus, he loved sports. Although I was employed full-time, I was actively involved at both of our sons schools. I'd been volunteering throughout my life and felt it was imperative, to teach my children the same. Since a kid, I had witnessed my Grandma use her gifts and talents to '**give back**', so it came naturally (to me). Rather than "telling" me the importance of volunteer work, my Grandma **showed** me, instead. There was a program in our city, in downtown Tulsa, that gave youth the opportunity (formerly headed by Mrs. Lynn Endres) to volunteer. I signed them both up, to give them a chance to become official 'Volunteer Youth Ambassadors'. So, my children and I would go to various places and give back together. During one summer, the program offered the 'Volunteer Ambassadors' the chance to meet the then Mayor (Judge LaFortune). It took place in South Tulsa, at the Hardesty Library, when it was still fairly new. The event was really neat and Tulsa's former Channel 8 News Anchor, Miss Yvonne Lewis (Harris) was even there. She did a short skit about the "Dos & Don'ts" at a job interview. It was actually Hilarious, because she seemingly came out of no where, with rollers in her hair and looking completely disheveled! Miss Lewis ran around the front of the room, as if she was clueless and seemingly lost. Obviously, this was her wonderful portrayal of what NOT to do at any interview (LOL!). Both of our sons had a great time, as well as others who were in attendance. So Justin and Quavi became fully immersed in their duties as Volunteers. They each enjoyed contributing to their community. Our oldest, Quavi even invited his best friend, Dillard to come along with us a few times. We each had productive, full schedules and busy days. However, in the imminent future, my Husband, our children and I-all four (4) of our lives would change and be greatly affected.

CHAPTER 3:

It Is, What It Is...

"You're going to wake-up one day and be unable to walk." I'm thinking to myself, WHOA...Hold-up! Wait, WHAT?! Those were the words uttered by the neurosurgeon, who I had been referred to by my Primary Care Physician (PCP). After performing an MRI, my then PCP sent me directly to a neurosurgeon-NOT a neurologist. So, whatever the report stated about my neck, it required surgery! Albeit, he was well-known, greatly respected, and "one of the best" in his field, surgery is STILL surgery. Shoot, that's all I could think of-surgery is surgery, No matter how you try to cut it (no pun intended, of course). I didn't care about his reputation or skills. Okay, in fairness, that's important too, but still...My mind was on anesthesia, getting cut, getting put "under"- You get my drift. Although my faith didn't wane during this, I was still very nervous. Truthfully, I was scared and what surgery might entail. I had A LOT of questions, as any married mother would! What about my boys? How will this affect my marriage? When will I be able to go back to work? Will my voice be the same? Ooh, will my voice be "deep"? Oh Lord, there'll be a scar! Will it be grotesque? I was beside myself with worry and angst. Thankfully, I had (still do) a level-headed and reassuring spouse. Joe **NEVER** doubted nor wavered, but remained steadfast in his optimism. The belief of, "It is, what it is and we'll get through it". As in any balanced relationship, I drew (my) strength from Joe's positivity and keen outlook. I was truly living Celine Dion's hit song, 'Because You Loved Me', in that moment. Needless to say, I had a successful surgery, with a prognosis of a twelve (12) week recovery period. However, I was better within a couple of weeks and ready to resume life, as regularly scheduled. So, I begged and pleaded with the surgeon, "to please release me." Finally, he did, with the stipulation that I would attend physical therapy, 'prn' (or as needed). By week four (4), I was at work and getting back to the swing of things. Thank God! However, in less than three (3) short months, life as my family and I knew it-would change, again...Sigh.

CHAPTER 4:

But God

Wow! This cannot be happening to us. Yet, again. Okay, let me rephrase my statement and retract. We are not any more special, than any other family nor are we invincible. Therefore, ANYTHING can happen to ANYONE of us and at ANY given time. However, Joe's injury was so out of left field and a rarity, in nature. I mean, I'd had major neck surgery less than three (3) months prior and we had just re-commenced our lives. Now, we were going from doctor to doctor to specialist to in-patient hospitalizations. Yes, as in 'plural', with an 'S'. After months of grueling appointments of poking and prodding Joe's limb, we were FINALLY given a correct diagnosis. Permanent nerve damage. The prognosis was not that great either-Unable to use that particular limb...**ever**. However, doctors are just human too. Even with the best intentions and a wealth of knowledge, as well as education, they are only people. Therefore, we respected their expertise but relied upon our Faith. We have always believed in the power of prayer and God. We had a relationship with Him (still do) and knew that He would heal my Husband. The journey was definitely Not an easy one. The first (1st) few years were difficult. Joe was in constant and horrendous pain, but he NEVER complained. He taught himself to do things with his other limb, regardless of the difficulty. Because Joe frequently visited doctors and specialists then needed to be hospitalized a few times, I took time away from work. I'd later makeup those hours around 2-3 in the morning and on some weekends. Since my work schedule was Monday through Friday, 8am to 5pm, I made arrangements ahead of time, so it could be improvised. My Mama, June was a big help, during that time. On the occasions that Joe was in the hospital, she and my then step-dad, Walt would keep our sons at their home then take them to school the following morning. Gratefully, their generosity allowed me to stay overnight with my Husband. If it were a weekday, I would leave early the next day and head to work. Because Joe and I now knew what we were facing with his injury, it was time to do something about it. We knew that God was on our side, during this process. So, it was time to do 'our part'. Joe just wanted relief from this consistent pain and aggravation. He went through physical rehabilitation, to no avail. He did water therapy, but that didn't help. His physician at the time, suggested ganglion blocks to "revive the nerves." However, after four (4) separate blocks, the doctor realized "there was too much scar tissue" and all four (4) ganglion blocks were unsuccessful. Joe went through various other procedures and treatments, but again nothing helped. After having a brutal laminectomy to help with the discomfort and the attempt to get some mobility in that limb, Joe was in recovery for a month. He was nearly bedridden, for a number of weeks. The performed laminectomy (through the back of the neck), was to "alleviate pressure on the nerves and decrease his symptoms, including numbness; tingling; throbbing and continuous pain." Since everything attempted at that point had failed, Joe went through another round of surgeries (a trial, a revision, and then an implantation of a spinal cord stimulator). Later, it had to be removed due to several issues of malfunctioning. The rehabilitation, procedures, and surgeries all went on for a period of years. Meanwhile, our sons were still actively playing sports and life continued. Those were some very trying and difficult times. Then, in the midst of Joe trying to get better from his injury, he became ill with pneumonia. It was during the holidays and mentally, emotionally taxing for all of us. It does something to the psyche, when one feels, you're going to lose someone that you love. Permanently. Regardless of everything that had taken place, I was Not going anywhere. I remained dedicated to my Husband's healing, for however long. We tried to maintain a sense of 'normalcy', within the boys' lives. I didn't want them to worry about their dad's health. It wasn't their responsibility and we wanted them to just be kids. I also didn't bother anyone with the specifics of what was going on. We only shared things with a few people like family (our Mothers and our Aunt Liz) and a handful of Good friends. My attitude was, "I appreciate your concern, but this is my Husband and I'll take care of him." You know that saying, "For better or for worse." Mainly, I knew people would have offered their support, had they been aware. However, I didn't want to be a bother. **<u>NOTE: Wrong</u>**! Be open AND honest about Your caregiving journey. Accept that help, especially when you know, it is genuine. Further, delegate tasks when applicable. The main purpose in my writing this, is to share My caregiving journey. More specifically, where I failed trying to do it all, Myself. Learn from 'Me' and take a different approach. Because, as a result of "doing it all", I kinda lost myself. Ironically, I neglected my own Self-Care. As humans, but more directly, as 'Women', we feel we can conquer the world! True, we're the givers of life and can multi-task like nobody's business. Give us a problem to solve, we will get a solution AND a resolution, **Period**. They don't say, "Girls Rule the World" for nothing. However, that 'Superwoman' mentality can be overwhelming, albeit exhausting. Besides, we Need each other and life, in all its complexities, are not meant to do so alone. Regardless who it is, male or female. We are Only human, so it is okay to not do it all by your lonesome. It Definitely has its consequences like burnout, fatigue, etc. But I'm getting ahead of myself and that's for another day, perhaps. So, my Husband got better and recovered from pneumonia, after almost dying from it. Although his limb didn't heal entirely, he learned to live with it. Joe has since taught himself, to primarily make usage of the other one. Throughout this ordeal, Joe has always maintained a positive attitude and vantage point. He **NEVER** felt sorry for himself or had a "woe is me", outlook. We credit everything to God's grace and mercy. He kept us, through it All. ALWAYS. We remained faithful, that His word was (Is) true, during each and every year our family experienced this. 'But God', He kept our family. Things weren't perfect and it was tough, but He was ALWAYS faithful to us. When doubt and worry crept in (because it did), we STILL Believed- remaining steadfast and devoted. When illness strikes, it can tear a couple and marriage a part. Statistically, the divorce rate is 75%, when one (1) spouse is chronically ill, according to a study from University of Michigan Researchers (a Time magazine article). Truthfully, dealing with things such as this and to this magnitude, it can be overwhelmingly frustrating and stressful in a relationship. And, though one is experiencing the "lows and valleys"-life is ongoing because time doesn't stop. Children are getting older and experiencing their own 'growing pains'. Jobs are only, but so patient. They are a business, after all. People (family; friends; employers; etc.) are dealing with their own "life issues". However, we refused to just "let life happen" without a fight. We tried our best to prioritize our home life balance:God and Family, first (1st). We continued to pray.... 'Together'. We continued our family nights....'Together'. Overall, we continued our lives....'Together'. No matter the circumstances, no matter how dismal, or the difficulty-we were dedicated, regardless. As a family, as well as a couple because "giving up" was NEVER an option. And candidly speaking, it really was ONLY through God's love, to have even an iota of the mental; Spiritual; physical and emotional capacity, to be able to endure (it all). The withal, to have the clarity of knowing 'Who' was (Is) in control. As a living witness throughout all of these trying times and Tribulations, I can testify that He is Real. 'But God'. Because had it not been for Him, we would not have been able to carry on.

CHAPTER 5:

About that Life

So he's on bended knee, anxious and ready to pop the question. Excitement is through the roof and the energy is contagious, infectious! The time has come and she finally answers in the affirmative, "YES, I'll marry you!" The cheers are endless and seemingly, never-ending. And then it hits everyone at once, "It's Party time and time to plan a wedding!" It's human nature to focus on the "good stuff" and ALL the wonderful things a wedding entails: the splendor, the beauty, the sweet beginnings. The aesthetics. Stunning bridal dress? Check. Beautiful decor? Check. Gorg wedding party AND attire? Check. Pretty cake? Check. Tasty and delicious food? Check. Awesome guest list, with a "just right" seating chart? Check. ALL of the elements of a "perfect wedding", huh? Well, what happens After the *Extravaganza*? Oh snap, that's right...oh my, the MARRIAGE! After all, this is the person you declared, "For richer or for poorer" to. If and when "in sickness and in health" comes (it can happen in short or long term marriages), what's next? Well, you do what needs to be done (whatever that means for you and your spouse). And I admit, our wedding was cool and our reception then after party was even better! But Married-life began AFTER the wedding and vows. In the situation we found ourselves in, after Joe's Medical predicament, it meant we had decisions to make. Ultimately, we chose to 'ride it out'…Together. We'd prayed about it and had faith, that we would come through on the other side. Period. Since I was still a parent and worked full-time, life had to be readjusted, compromises had to be made, as well as sacrifices. Because Joe was going to a multitude of doctors and specialists that didn't always share information with the other, I made up a diary-style journal. I like organization and order, so I wrote it to include ALL of Joe's pertinent medical data. For other Caregivers reading this, I learned early-on how helpful this made EVERYTHING, for me and the doctors/specialists. I included a 'Table of Contents', plus various sections for the physician, their field of specialty, as well as their demographics (address; office contact; fax numbers; et cetera). In addition, there were areas for insurance information; applicable health conditions; personal data (weight, height, pharmacy, etc) and a Miscellaneous/MISC. section. Of course, this was years before 'My Chart' was on the market and a patient could view their medical history, online. This journal made it easy to have everything needed, at each and every visit and in one (1) place. It was so beneficial, that I created one for other

Caregivers or anyone else who need and want to keep <u>All</u> of their medical health history organized. It simplified Joe's appointments. For instance, if an authorization needed to be scheduled with a specialist, I would share their demographics with the Physician's office staff, on the spot. Therefore, it made the referral process a quick, simple, and convenient one, for all parties involved. Instead of writing down a list of Joe's medications, when he went to visit a doctor, I would just give them a photocopy from the journal I had made. I kept it up-to-date (with dosage amounts; milligrams; reasons for the medicine; et cetera) and legible, so that check-in and time in the waiting room were shortened. There were small "tricks" such as these, to make my caregiving life a lot less complicated. Although it wasn't always easy, I kept my **Why's** in perspective, the reasons that I was My Husband's Caregiver. No, I wasn't "obligated" nor did Joe make me feel, as such. He had ALWAYS taken care of me and our family, so I did what was in my heart to reciprocate. The Vow I made, to love and care for him, "in sickness and in health" was what I intended to **DO**. So my fellow Caregivers, I'm sending You positivity, good vibes, and prayers on your Own caregiving pilgrimages and adventures. At the end of the day, you have EVERYTHING you need, to aid in your loved one's care inside of you. Love+Empathy+Heart, equals 'Giving' the Best Care, as their personal Caretaker…YOU.

ACT 3

Ms. Carver's Story

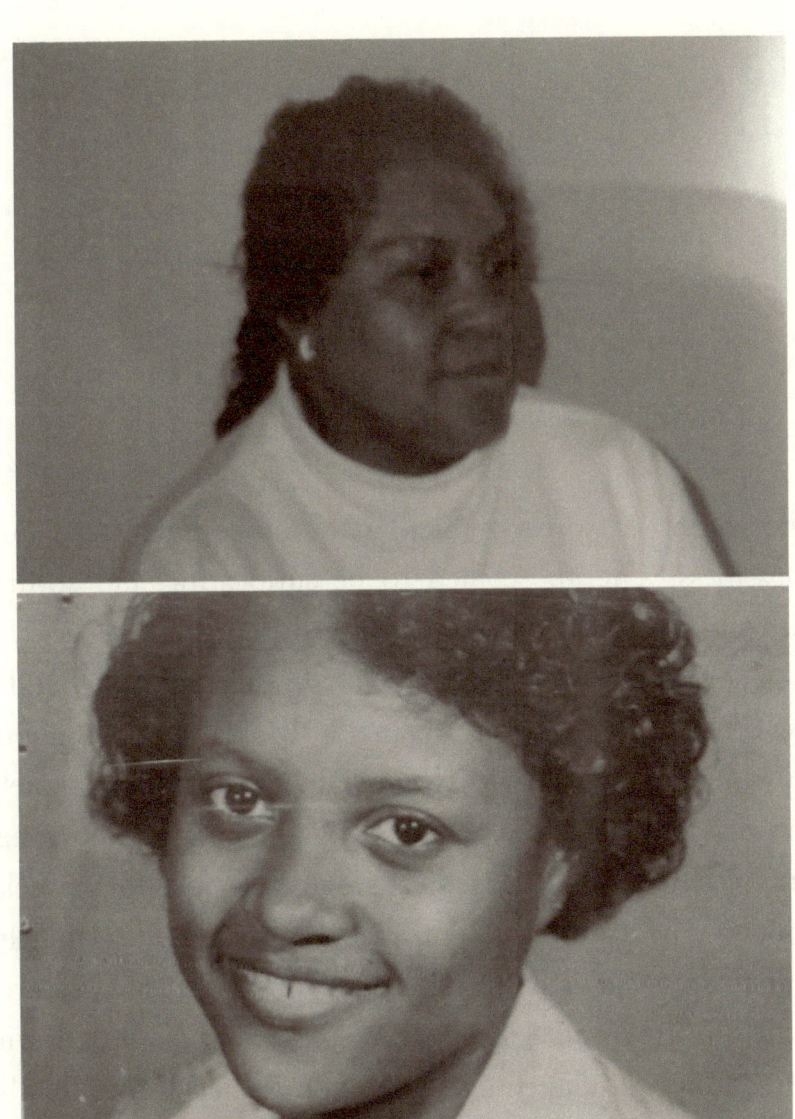

Pretty Lady: My Mother-in-Law, Ms. JoE.C.

CHAPTER 1:

No News Is Good News

The room was dreary, thick with foreboding dread and uneasiness. The air seemed to be suffocating and stifling with obvious undertones of fear and apprehensiveness. I'd been sitting with my Husband, Joe; his brother, Billy; and a few other relatives, while we anxiously awaited news about my mother-in-law's health. Ms. EllaJo Carver, (affectionately known as 'Nanny' and 'Aunt Jo' by her Grand's and other family) had endured a Medical emergency, just a few weeks prior and was admitted into the hospital. Unfortunately, at that time, she was still under the hospital's care. Forever etched in my mind, I vividly remember that gloomy day in 2013. It was Sunday, June 16th and on Father's Day. Usually, I'd cook or me and our children would celebrate Joe, by taking him to dinner after church services. However, the only plans we (Joe and I) had that day, was to go to the hospital after church then "find something to eat", later. Joe had been there all of the previous day and his Mama was the Only thing on his mind…his **ONLY** agenda. Understandably. So, we proceeded to church. Sometime before services ended, Joe received a call from the hospital. The message relayed was somewhat vague, but "urgent"! We hurriedly rushed there, without hesitation. Thankfully, our Pastor and First Lady (Pastors Scotty and Dena Baler) at the time, along with our close-knit church family knew that Ms. Carver had been hospitalized. Further, it wasn't necessary to explain something we were still unsure of ourselves. We knew they had been praying for her, as well as for our family. Although Joe didn't yet know what had happened so quickly with her health status, he called his sister and brother (who both lived locally) to get to the hospital. My Husband has a really easy-going, laid-back personality for anyone who knows him, but I could see the turmoil in his eyes. He didn't vocalize his anguish, but sadness registered throughout his body language. I could sense his pain, because it was so detectable and palpable. It scared me to witness him looking so forlorn and still NOT know exactly what we were "walking into". We weren't aware of the soon devastation at the time, but we knew one thing…it wasn't going to be "Good" news.

CHAPTER 2:

The Fragile State of Life

Previous to this life-changing Father's Day and weeks prior, Ms. Carver had had plenty of family and friends come to see her. For one, my sister-in-law Charlene had gone to the hospital and braided our mother-in-law's hair, while they chatted. Later, family out of Kansas City had come for the weekend to visit. No one could have predicted how quickly her health would eventually deteriorate. Gratefully, she was able to share laughs, heartfelt and memorable conversations with her love ones, before life took such a drastic turn. So, we arrived at the hospital and met-up with Joe's two (2) siblings (the other 2 lived out of state) and my mama June, then checked-in to see Ms. Carver. After our visit, additional family members had come to the hospital. By this time, Ms. Carver's Attending Physician had pulled Joe aside, along with his brother, Billy and their sister, Carla to talk in confidence. Our niece, Tawny walked with us, as we all followed behind the Physician. We knew this situation was serious, so I walked hand in hand with my Husband. We were not quite sure of their mother's prognosis, but keenly aware that it was crucial. The doctor led us into a room and excused herself, momentarily. There we sat and each stewing in our own thoughts, in angst. The energy was somber and everyone was trying to remain calm, level-headed. Although indecisive about what this conversation would entail, we continued to sit there and waited patiently. Minutes seemed like hours, but it wasn't long before the doctor came back into the room to talk with us, expectantly. Although I don't recall everything about that moment, what I do remember stood out to me. It was as if the doctor had a lisp, who spoke in a foreign tongue with an unknown dialect (none of which was true, of course). She seemed to be talking in a language that was unfamiliar to me and in slow motion. I started talking to myself like, "Did she just say Hospice Care?" Wait, wait, wait…back up, now WHAT now?! It seemed what little oxygen that remained, had been completely sucked out of the room. It was like having an out of body experience hearing this, honestly. The realization and severity of those 2 words ('Hospice Care') were like a jolt of something indescribable. I remember Carla bursting into tears, while Tawny comforted her. I felt powerless, so helpless, as to what to do next. Joe and Billy were both trying to make sense of the huge "crater", that the doctor had just dropped. They tried to decipher what all of this meant. To say they were flabbergasted, would be an understatement.

They looked so despondent. My normally "cool as a fan" and kind-hearted Husband, looked so perplexed and crest-fallen. My heart immediately broke. I hurt for myself, my children and all of Ms. Carver's grandchildren, as well as the countless other loved ones. But I was especially heartbroken for her Children, all five (5) of them because this was their 'Mother'. And we only get one (1) of those in this lifetime. It was just too much and too soon, to digest such an enormous blow. Plus, the news still needed to be broken to her other two (2) daughters, Belinda and Shelly. They lived in a different state, along with other immediate family members of Ms. Carver's like additional grandchildren, great grand's, etc. Sure, we knew she was ill. However, we had remained prayerful and optimistic that she would get better then be released from the hospital. So how did we go from that to this finality of 'Hospice Care'? It just seemed, so Unreal. It felt like it was far too much to bear. Then a sobering reality hit, how fragile life is…

CHAPTER 3:

At the End of the Day

You know, they say your life flashes before your eyes when it's "your time to go." However true that may be, I started having glimpses of the nearly 20 years that my mother-in-law had been in my life. During that timeframe in 2013, I had been married to her youngest son for nineteen (19) years and we had had two (2) sons. Ms. Carver's presence and influence were prevalent in both of my pregnancies. She was never the kind of mother-in-law and grandmother (Nanny) to butt into your business or offer unsolicited advice. No, she'd offer sage wisdom, at the right intervals or at the precise moments that they were warranted. She was NEVER "meddlesome" or overbearing in our relationship and ultimate marriage. I greatly appreciated her authenticity. Ms. Carver minded her own business. However, she would speak her peace about a situation then be done with it. Over the many years I was her daughter-in-law, we had some good laughs and times. One thing Joe, Ms. Carver, and I loved to do was go "junking" together. Not everyone can get into going from garage sale to yard sale, just to find the right bargains. But it was something that we enjoyed doing together. I can still hear her saying certain things because of something goofy I did or said. I crack up laughing now, thinking of her little sayings. I also look back at the friendship that she and my grandma developed, over the years and smile. My grandma was older than Ms. Carver by a few years. Though they were different in many ways, they had mutual respect and a fondness of the other. I liked their comradery, too. When our sons were in elementary school, they both played a variety of sports. So we would get Joe's mother together with my grandma and we'd all go to our boys T-ball, baseball, and soccer games (depending who was playing). It would be hilarious watching and listening to both grandma and great-grandma. Those two (2) would literally "coach" the kids from the sidelines. They'd tell the kids to go the right way on the field "this time." LOL! They would themselves laugh because the kids would throw the ball elsewhere or run the wrong way on the field. It was just funny being at some of our children's games with my grandma and mother-in-law. But more than anything, I am so happy they BOTH got the chance to meet their grandsons and great-grandsons, respectfully. Those are fond memories that Joe and I still talk about today. And years later when Joe and I became the Primary Caregiver to my grandma, Ms. Carver was right there. On one (1) occasion, she stepped-in and helped me with her nightly duties. Later that same evening, an ambulance had to be called for grandma and Ms. Carver remained with me. She could tell I was trying to be strong and "keep it together" due to my grandma's health crisis. She kindly moved me aside and went directly into 'Nurse mode'. Both My husband and mother-in-law teamed up and assisted my grandma. While Joe talked with 911, he and Ms. Carver stayed by her side.

They never once left her, until my grandma was safely inside the ambulance. I have NEVER forgotten such a selfless act. Ms. Carver sensed that I was on the verge of tears and barely able to compose myself. She knew me and could tell that I was going into shock. It was completely devastating. She was also keenly aware how much my grandma meant to me and how close I was to her. Ms. Carver never once said a word to me. Instead, she immediately went into action and continued to keep my grandma alert. Time was of the essence and my mother-in-law wasted none of it. Not even for a nanosecond. So all of these thoughts floated in my mind's eye, at the hospital that fateful day. 'Hospice Care'. Unbelievable. The plan had been once she was discharged, she would then come live with us. We had recently moved from an apartment to a house, so Ms. Carver could come home with Joe, our youngest son, Justin and I. Our oldest son, Quavi was in college out of state. Further, before she had fallen ill, Ms. Carver, Joe, and I had discussed her living with the three (3) of us. If need be, we decided that we would hire a Nurse on an "as needed basis." The transition would have been an easy one. At the beginning of our courtship, I had lived with Ms. Carver and Joe. So, this process would have been no different. It's what family does and are "supposed" to do for one another. My grandma **ALWAYS** put family first (1st), so this was ingrained and instilled within me. Plus, as long as Joe had breath in his body and was alive on God's green earth, his mama would **NEVER** be turned away, ever! So, it was decided that Ms. Carver would come home to live with us through Hospice Care services. Unfortunately, in most US States, the prognosis for a Hospice Care Patient is 6-12 months *(per the Hospice agency)*. Gratefully, she would be surrounded by love and loved on by family. Because at the end of the day, it's about being thankful for even the seemingly "small" blessings and "tiny" glimmers of hope. At that point, we were just Thankful that she was still…Alive.

CHAPTER 4:

The Matriarch

A retired widower, who lived a life full with fierce independence and strength. A daughter, the youngest of only two (2) girls, out of a combined thirteen (13) siblings (children). A mother of five (5) adult children. A grandmother ('Nanny') of fifteen (15). A great, great-great, and great-great-great grandmother of a multitude of grand. An aunt. A cousin. A sister. A niece. A daughter-in-law. A friend. A listener. A sister-in-law. A confidante. A gardener. A Mother-in-law. A seamstress. A baker. A healer. A gourmet food connoisseur & cook. A caretaker. A pastry chef. A nurse. A truth-giver. A gatekeeper of secrets. A Woman who embodied and embraced Traditional values, but understood the fabric of today's society, without succumbing to its current "trends." A Classic beauty, who loved and cherished her family with an obvious determination and drive. Ms. EllaJo Carver had been so much, to so many and for so long, that it was only proper to give her the same in return. She deserved our love; our appreciation; our patience; and our diligence. The Matriarch. A daughter that helped care for her own mother. A dutiful wife, who was the epitome of her other half's 'Helpmate'. A sister who also assisted in the care of All of her now-deceased brothers. A mother, who wasn't just that in name, but also in action and reality. Ms. EllaJo was **All** of the aforementioned and more. If there were ever a time to 'Honor & Cherish' The Matriarch, *("the head of a family-a mother over her descendants",* paraphrased definition of 'matriarch' on google). Well, this was THAT time. It was 'Her' time, Ms. EllaJo Carver's. The Matriarch.

CHAPTER 5:

Dignity, Love, and Respect: FULL STOP

You know something that I've learned in life? Sometimes, you don't know your own strength, until you've encountered and actually lived an experience. Specifically, a 'life and death' situation. In fact, and personally speaking, let me rephrase that sentiment. I did NOT know my 'Own' strength, until going through such an ordeal. I was absolutely unfamiliar with anything quite like Hospice. It was a tough predicament to endure, both mentally and emotionally. I mean, how does one ever process something of this magnitude? How do you even prepare life, knowing that a Person you love and care for, will no longer be here? The inevitable will soon come to pass and you have to helplessly watch them… die. These were the many thoughts running rampantly in my mind. However morbid, macabre, and ghastly this way of thinking is, it's honest. I am Human and internally my emotions were thwarted everywhere. I know no one likes to think about death, let alone talk about it. But I want to share 'My' personal journey to help another person who may be going through this now. In writing this particular chapter, I am sharing my initial frame of mind. I was frightened; sad; confused; grieving and just a ball of emotions. However, at the forefront of everything mentioned, I knew I needed to be strong for my husband, Joe. Yes, I was sorrowful, but this was his Mama. A mama, who he had a very close relationship with and who he loved extensively, dearly. A mother whom he shared with four (4) siblings, who had their own loving relationships with their mother. So, I made a decision right then and there in that "little room" at the hospital, in whatever capacity Joe and his siblings needed me, I'd take care of my mother-in-law, Ms. EllaJo Carver. It was nice when various family members came to visit with her. Some lived in different places in OK, while others came in from Wichita, KS. In between this activity, I helped the Hospice Care Nurse keep Ms. Carver comfortable; give prescribed medications; bathe her; etc. Respectfully, I took myself completely out of the equation because it was NOT about 'me'. However long that we still had Ms. EllaJo in our lives, it was all about 'HER'. Period. Had the roles been reversed, I knew she would have been right by Joe's side, her son and helped him with my care. Even to just sit and visit with me. So, I put on my "big girl panties" (as the saying goes), along with my grief and placed them on the backburner. Then did what ANY daughter-in-law, would have done for their Mother-in-law: I cared for her with Dignity, Love, and Respect. FULL STOP.

CHAPTER 6:

Never…Ever

It was early, just past dawn and the day had started out beautifully. The sun shone brightly, against the backdrop of a clear, blue skyline. It was June, so Summertime was in full swing. The birds were chirping away, while a duo of blue jays chased the other through the vastness of trees. They seemed to play tag, right outside of Ms. Carver's window, going from limb to branch in quick succession. Their playful banter seemed so carefree, so cheery, and so light. It was the complete and stark opposite of the interior at our home. With the exception of Gospel music playing softly in Ms. EllaJo's room, there was an eerie silence. Although we didn't know the dreaded and appointed time, we knew that 'The Time' was near. June 26, 2013. The birthday of our First Lady at the time, Sister (Pastor) Dena Baler. And just the previous day, my mama, June had turned a year older too. Both days were met with somber melancholy. Sister Baler and her husband, our Pastor Scotty Baler were vacationing with family, to rightfully celebrate another year of her life. Even still, The Baler's took time from their schedules and day, to pray with and for us, over the phone. They extended their genuine encouragement, love, and support to our family. The Chaplain also came to our home and offered the same comfort. He had prayed over Ms. Carver, as well, knowing her transition would be soon. Justin was over a friend's and Quavi was in town due to summer break, at his friend's too. Joe and I had checked on the other because neither of us had had much, if any sleep. Then hours later and on the same morning, my Mother-in-law of nearly twenty (20) years in the course of this time-frame, passed away. Sleeping peacefully, Ms. EllaJo took her last breath, while the blue jays ascended in the air. And though we knew the imminent future and "what was to come", it's still NEVER easy to lose a loved one and say a Final goodbye…Ever.

CHAPTER 7:

Remembered, Always

Today, nearly ten (10) years later Ms. EllaJo Carver's memory is still alive. Though she is missed immensely, we still cherish her memory. She was the last of her siblings to transition, so her loss is ever present. There's an unspoken sadness and gloominess that is present in our home, when Ms. EllaJo's birthday comes around each April. I can feel the slight shift in my husband's energy, who is usually good-humored and cheerful. Without audibly saying anything, after being married nearly thirty (30) years, I can see the somber intensity in Joe's eyes. I sense and can feel the heaviness, knowing his heart. He doesn't "complain", rather deals with the enormity of the occasion in his own way. As I'm sure the rest of her children and grandchildren do. Since Ms. Carver's passing, our Aunt Violet (who's birthday is close to hers) and other close relatives check on Joe, especially during his mom's birthday month. Our cousin Danielle, who he talks to frequently, always call during that time. Her mom, Our Aunt Willa also shared a birthday close to Ms. Carver's. So, they offer comfort to the other, while memorializing their mothers. Although Ms. EllaJo is no longer here in flesh, we keep her likeness alive, by sharing who she was and what she (still) means, to the new generation. As the famous and popular saying goes, "Gone but NEVER forgotten", because Ms. EllaJo Carver's legacy lives on. Through the lives of her many descendants, her footprint and landscape on this earth will be eternally cemented, due to their vast and varying contributions to this world. She would be proud, in fact "tinkled pink" for the young lives she had not had the chance to meet. These lives, who are continuing her lineage. One (1) thing is for sure and two (2) is for certain, Ms. EllaJo will be Forever remembered. Always. All of the things that made the woman, Who she was-her essence; her existence; her life; her mark…Always, Remembered.

Lessons Caring for a Hospice Care Patient or Incapacitated Loved One:

(1) Remember, it's about them-NOT you.

(2) **Hearing** is the last sense that leaves, when a Person is dying.
  A. Keep Gospel, Classical, or (**Any**) Soft music playing in their background.
  B. Talk to your loved one, in a gentle tone & **Don't** ignore them because they can hear You.

(3) Find a reputable 'Hospice Care' agency, if they're not going to live with family. Even if loved one will be living with family, connect with a Great agency.
  A. The Agency is (usually) good about letting the family be involved in Loved One's care.
  B. 'Hospice' is there to 'Guide & Assist' You with your Loved One.

(4) Surround your Loved One(s) with family, in intervals, as to NOT overwhelm the Patient.

(5) Shower them with love and be patient in **their** process. They may be tired and sleepy a lot, so don't take things personally and be Mindful, of this.

(6) Sometimes, it may be beneficial to just sit with them, Quietly.

(7) Read to your Loved One(s) like the Bible; their favorite book; something in relation to their religion; a Motivational story; a devotion; et cetera.

(8) Pray over them, if too difficult for the Caregiver, have a Chaplain (usually through the Hospice agency); a Priest; a Pastor; et cetera., to do so.

(9) Follow **ALL** medication instructions and protocols, according to agency.
A. Make certain meds are given appropriately and in its **EXACT** dosage and/or form.
B. Remember, keep a Detailed time-line (date; Rx/ prescriptions; milligrams; Signature/initials; et cetera) when logging-in Patient's Medical information and medicine, through Hospice agency *keeps things organized for the Shift-Nurses, as well as for the Patient's family*

(10) Visit with your Loved One as OFTEN as possible, because you don't know their end.

(11) Take time away, just as frequently, as to NOT get overwhelmed or over-emotional (your Loved One can **STILL** Hear you).

(12) Stay hydrated, well-rested, and nourished to keep Your strength & energy.

(13) Be gentle, but thorough during All of their bathing times.

(14) Keep your Loved One's space sanitary and uncluttered, at **All** times.

(15) Make sure their clothing is clean and they have 'Light & Airy' clothes available.

(16) Last, but NOT least: Take Care of Your **OWN** Self-Care management, whatever that entails for You (yoga; exercise; prayer; daily affirmations; et cetera). It is just as Important, as the Care that you give to your Love One(s).

www.ingramcontent.com/pod-product-compliance
Lightning Source LLC
Chambersburg PA
CBHW030031250526
45464CB00025B/1103